Reviving Traditional Herbal Remedies for Today's Health:

The Lost Guide Book of Herbal

Natural Remedies

Rediscovering Nature's

Healing Wisdom

Contents

Introduction

In the bustling cacophony of modern life, where synthetic solutions often overshadow the natural, there exists a timeless wisdom waiting to be rediscovered—the ancient art of herbal medicine. Welcome to "Reviving Traditional Herbal Remedies for Today's Health: The

Lost Guide Book of Herbal Natural Remedies Rediscovering Nature's Healing Wisdom."

In the pursuit of progress, we've sometimes overlooked the profound healing potential that lies within the embrace of nature. Yet, the remedies that sustained humanity for millennia still hold relevance in our quest for holistic well-being. This book is an invitation to journey back to our

roots, to explore the forgotten

pathways of herbal wisdom, and

to rekindle our relationship with

the healing power of plants.

The Lost Wisdom: Rediscovering Herbal Remedies

Embedded within the fabric of

history, herbal medicine has been

a steadfast companion to humanity's journey through time. From the ancient civilizations of Mesopotamia to the traditional healers of Africa and the indigenous tribes of the Americas, every culture has cultivated its unique relationship with the flora of the earth. Yet, as civilizations advanced and the allure of modernity beckoned, the profound knowledge of herbal remedies began to fade into obscurity, relegated to the annals of forgotten lore.

The Relevance of Traditional Herbal Medicine Today

In an age characterized by the resurgence of holistic living and a growing disillusionment with synthetic remedies, the time is ripe for a renaissance of herbal medicine. As we confront the complexities of modern health challenges—from chronic stress and immune disorders to environmental toxins and antibiotic resistance—we find ourselves turning once again to the wisdom of our ancestors for guidance. In the face of uncertainty, the reassuring embrace of nature's pharmacy offers a beacon of hope—a pathway to healing that honors the interconnectedness of mind, body, and spirit.

Understanding the Power of Plants in Healing

At the heart of herbal medicine lies a profound respect for the innate intelligence of the natural world. Each plant, with its unique combination of phytochemicals and therapeutic properties, offers a gift of healing waiting to be unlocked. From the humble chamomile flower to the mighty ginseng root, the diversity of plant medicine reflects the boundless creativity of the earth itself. By harnessing the power of plants in synergy with our own innate healing capacity, we embark on a journey of transformation—a journey towards greater vitality, resilience, and harmony.

In the pages that follow, we will delve into the rich tapestry of herbal medicine, exploring ancient traditions, rediscovering forgotten remedies, and empowering ourselves to embrace a more holistic approach to health and wellness. Together, let us embark on a journey of rediscovery—a journey that leads us back to the timeless wisdom encoded within the leaves, roots, and flowers of the natural world.

Welcome to the lost guidebook of herbal natural remedies—where ancient wisdom meets modern healing, and nature's healing wisdom is rediscovered.

Chapter 1: Foundations of Herbal Medicine

In the vast expanse of human history, the roots of herbal medicine run deep, intertwining with the very essence of our existence. In this chapter, we will embark on a journey through time, tracing the lineage of herbal medicine from its ancient origins to its modern-day resurgence. We will explore the foundational principles that underpin this ancient healing art and delve into the scientific insights that validate its efficacy.

A Brief History of Herbal Medicine

To understand herbal medicine is to journey back through the annals of time, to the dawn of human civilization itself. From the earliest hunter-gatherers who roamed the earth to the sophisticated societies of antiquity, our ancestors looked to the plants that surrounded them for sustenance, shelter, and healing. In every corner of the globe, indigenous cultures developed their unique systems of herbal medicine, passing down their knowledge through oral traditions, written texts, and the healing hands of wise elders. We will trace the evolution of herbal medicine through the ages, from the ancient wisdom of Ayurveda and Traditional Chinese Medicine to the herbal lore of Europe and the Americas.

The Science Behind Herbal Remedies

While herbal medicine has its roots in ancient wisdom, its efficacy is increasingly being validated by modern science. In this section, we will explore the biochemical mechanisms that underlie the therapeutic actions of medicinal plants. From the anti-inflammatory properties of turmeric to the antimicrobial effects of garlic, we will uncover the pharmacological secrets hidden within nature's pharmacy. Through the lens of chemistry, pharmacology, and physiology, we will gain a deeper appreciation for the complex interactions between plants and the human body, shedding light on why herbal remedies continue to hold relevance in our modern world.

Principles of Herbal Healing

At the heart of herbal medicine lies a set of guiding principles that inform its practice. Whether rooted in ancient traditions or modern research, these principles serve as the foundation upon which effective herbal treatment is built. We will explore concepts such as the doctrine of signatures, which holds that plants resemble the organs they are meant to heal, and the concept of energetics, which seeks to balance the body's vital forces through the use of specific herbs. By understanding these principles, we gain insight into the art and science of herbal healing, empowering us to harness the full potential of nature's bounty in our quest for health and wellness.

As we journey deeper into the realm of herbal medicine, let us remember that our exploration is not merely an intellectual exercise but a sacred pilgrimage—an invitation to reconnect with the timeless wisdom encoded within the plants that surround us. In the chapters that follow, we will continue our quest for knowledge, uncovering the hidden treasures of herbal medicine and embracing a more holistic approach to health and healing.

Chapter 2: The Lost Herbal Remedies

In the vast tapestry of herbal medicine, there exists a treasure trove of remedies waiting to be rediscovered. In this chapter, we will embark on a journey through time and space, exploring the forgotten pathways of herbal wisdom and unearthing the hidden gems of traditional medicine from cultures around the world.

Exploring Forgotten Herbal Traditions

Throughout history, herbal medicine has flourished in diverse cultures, each with its unique traditions and practices. From the ancient civilizations of Mesopotamia and Egypt to the indigenous tribes of Africa, Asia, and the Americas, every corner of the globe has cultivated its rich botanical heritage. Yet, as the tides of time swept across the land, many of these herbal traditions were lost or suppressed, their knowledge relegated to the shadows of history. In this section, we will shine a light on these forgotten traditions, uncovering the herbal remedies that sustained our ancestors for generations.

Rediscovering Ancient Herbal Texts

Embedded within the pages of ancient manuscripts lie the

secrets of herbal medicine, waiting to be deciphered by those who dare to seek them out. In this section, we will journey into the archives of history, exploring the wisdom preserved in texts such as the Ebers Papyrus, the Yellow Emperor's Inner Canon, and the writings of Hippocrates and Dioscorides. Through the eyes of these ancient scribes, we will gain insight into the medicinal properties of plants, the art of herbal preparation, and the principles of healing that have stood the test of time.

Unearthing Hidden Remedies from Around the World

Beyond the confines of written texts lie a wealth of oral traditions, passed down through generations by healers, shamans, and wise women. In this section, we will travel to the far corners of the earth, seeking out the herbal remedies that have sustained indigenous cultures for millennia. From the healing chants of the Maori to the sacred plant ceremonies of the Amazon rainforest, we will bear witness to the profound connection between people and plants and the wisdom that arises from living in harmony with the natural world.

As we journey deeper into the realm of lost herbal remedies, let us approach with humility and reverence, honoring the wisdom of our ancestors and the sacred bond between humanity and the plant kingdom. In the chapters that follow, we will continue our quest to revive these ancient traditions, bringing their healing wisdom into the light once more.

Chapter 3: Building Your Herbal Toolkit

In the pursuit of herbal wellness, preparation is key. In this chapter, we will explore the essential tools, techniques, and practices necessary for building your herbal toolkit. From selecting and harvesting medicinal plants to creating your own herbal apothecary, this chapter will empower you to embark on your journey with confidence and clarity.

Selecting and Harvesting Medicinal Plants

The journey of herbal medicine begins with the selection of the finest botanical specimens. In this section, we will delve into the art and science of plant identification, learning to recognize the distinctive features of medicinal herbs in their natural habitat. From the gentle curve of a leaf to the vibrant hue of a flower, each plant offers clues to its identity and therapeutic potential. We will also discuss the ethical considerations of wildcrafting and the importance of sustainable harvesting practices in preserving our precious plant allies for future generations.

Essential Tools and Equipment for Herbal Preparation

To transform raw plant material into potent remedies requires a set of essential tools and equipment. In this section, we will explore the must-have items for your herbal toolkit, from mortar and pestle to herbal presses and tincture bottles. We will discuss the importance of quality craftsmanship and materials in ensuring the efficacy and safety of your herbal preparations, as well as practical tips for sourcing and caring for your equipment.

Creating Your Herbal Apothecary

Your herbal apothecary is the heart and soul of your healing practice—a sacred space where plants are transformed into medicine and wisdom is distilled into remedies. In this section, we will guide you through the process of setting up your own herbal apothecary, from organizing your workspace to stocking your shelves with essential herbs, oils, and extracts. We will also discuss the principles of herbal formulation and the art of creating custom blends tailored to individual needs and preferences.

As you embark on your journey to build your herbal toolkit, remember that the path of herbal medicine is one of lifelong learning and discovery. With dedication, patience, and a deep reverence for the plants that sustain us, you will cultivate a rich and rewarding relationship with the world of herbal healing.

Chapter 4: Herbal Remedies for Common Ailments

In this chapter, we will explore a variety of herbal remedies for addressing common ailments that affect our everyday lives. From digestive disorders to respiratory issues and stress-related conditions, we will discover how herbal medicine offers gentle yet effective solutions for promoting health and well-being.

Natural Solutions for Digestive Disorders

The digestive system is the foundation of health, and herbal medicine offers a wealth of remedies for supporting its optimal function. In this section, we will explore herbs such as ginger, peppermint, and chamomile, which can soothe digestive discomfort, relieve bloating and gas, and promote healthy digestion. We will also discuss the role of bitter herbs in stimulating digestive juices and enhancing nutrient absorption, as well as the importance of dietary and lifestyle factors in maintaining digestive wellness.

Herbal Treatments for Respiratory Health

From the common cold to chronic respiratory conditions such as asthma and bronchitis, herbal medicine offers a variety of remedies for supporting respiratory health. In this section, we will explore herbs such as elderberry, thyme, and eucalyptus, which have expectorant, antimicrobial, and anti-inflammatory properties that can help alleviate coughs, congestion, and inflammation in the respiratory tract. We will also discuss the use of steam inhalations, herbal teas, and chest rubs as natural ways to promote respiratory comfort and ease breathing.

Soothing Herbs for Stress and Anxiety

In our fast-paced modern world, stress and anxiety have become increasingly common concerns that can take a toll on our physical, mental, and emotional well-being. In this section, we will explore herbs such as lemon balm, passionflower, and holy basil, which have nervine and adaptogenic properties that can help calm the mind, reduce tension, and support the body's response to stress. We will also discuss the role of lifestyle practices such as mindfulness, relaxation techniques, and herbal baths in promoting relaxation and emotional balance.

As we explore these herbal remedies for common ailments, let us remember that the key to effective healing lies not only in the remedies themselves but also in the holistic approach to health and wellness that herbal medicine embodies. By nourishing the body, mind, and spirit with the healing gifts of nature, we can cultivate a deeper sense of vitality, resilience, and harmony in

our lives.

Chapter 5: Herbs for Holistic Wellness

In this chapter, we will delve into the realm of holistic wellness and explore a diverse array of herbs that support balance and vitality in body, mind, and spirit. From hormone regulation to immune support and cognitive enhancement, we will discover how herbal medicine offers comprehensive solutions for optimizing overall well-being.

Balancing Hormones Naturally

Hormonal balance is essential for overall health and vitality, yet many factors in modern life can disrupt the delicate equilibrium of our endocrine system. In this section, we will explore herbs such as chasteberry, black cohosh, and dong quai, which have been traditionally used to support hormonal balance in women. We will also discuss the role of adaptogenic herbs such as ashwagandha and rhodiola in helping the body adapt to stress and maintain hormonal harmony.

Boosting Immunity with Herbal Support

A strong immune system is our body's first line of defense against illness and infection, and herbal medicine offers a wealth of remedies for bolstering immune function. In this section, we will explore herbs such as echinacea, elderberry, and astragalus, which have immune-stimulating and antiviral properties that can help prevent and combat infections. We will also discuss the importance of lifestyle factors such as diet, sleep, and stress management in supporting immune health and resilience.

Promoting Mental Clarity and Focus

In our fast-paced, information-saturated world, maintaining mental clarity and focus is essential for productivity, creativity, and overall well-being. In this section, we will explore herbs such as ginkgo biloba, bacopa, and gotu kola, which have cognitive-enhancing properties that can help improve memory, concentration, and mental acuity. We will also discuss the role of mindfulness practices, brain-boosting nutrients, and herbal teas in supporting brain health and cognitive function.

As we explore these herbs for holistic wellness, let us remember that true health is not merely the absence of disease but a state of vibrant vitality and harmony in body, mind, and spirit. By embracing the wisdom of herbal medicine and incorporating these healing herbs into our daily lives, we can cultivate a deeper sense of well-being and thrive in our modern world.

Chapter 6: Herbal Remedies for Skin and Hair

Our skin and hair are not only reflections of our inner health but also our outer beauty. In this chapter, we will explore the wonders of herbal remedies for nurturing healthy skin and vibrant hair. From soothing irritation to enhancing radiance, herbal medicine offers a natural and effective approach to skincare and haircare.

Nourishing Herbs for Healthy Skin

Healthy skin begins with proper nourishment and care. In this section, we will explore a variety of herbs such as calendula, lavender, and aloe vera, which have moisturizing, anti-inflammatory, and healing properties that can soothe irritation, promote cell regeneration, and restore balance to the skin. We will also discuss the role of herbal infusions, oils, and balms in creating a personalized skincare routine that nurtures and protects the skin.

Herbal Treatments for Common Skin Conditions

From acne and eczema to psoriasis and rosacea, herbal medicine offers gentle yet effective remedies for a variety of common skin conditions. In this section, we will explore herbs such as tea tree oil, chamomile, and burdock root, which have antibacterial, anti-inflammatory, and detoxifying properties that can help alleviate symptoms and promote healing. We will also discuss the importance of addressing underlying imbalances and triggers to achieve long-term skin health and vitality.

Enhancing Hair Health with Herbal Solutions

Our hair is a reflection of our overall health and vitality, and herbal medicine offers a holistic approach to hair care that nourishes the scalp, strengthens the hair shaft, and enhances shine and manageability. In this section, we will explore herbs such as rosemary, nettle, and horsetail, which have tonic, revitalizing, and conditioning properties that can promote healthy hair growth, reduce breakage, and restore luster to dull, damaged hair. We will also discuss the role of scalp massage, herbal rinses, and nourishing hair masks in maintaining optimal hair health and beauty.

As we explore these herbal remedies for skin and hair, let us remember that beauty is not merely skin deep but a reflection of our inner vitality and well-being. By embracing the wisdom of herbal medicine and treating our skin and hair with care and reverence, we can nourish our bodies from the inside out and radiate beauty and vitality for

years to come.

Chapter 7: Herbal Remedies for Women's Health

Women's health encompasses a diverse array of physiological and emotional needs throughout the various stages of life. In this chapter, we will explore the gentle yet powerful herbal remedies that support women's health, from menstrual wellness to hormonal balance and beyond.

Supporting Menstrual Health Naturally

The menstrual cycle is a natural and essential aspect of women's reproductive health, yet many women experience discomfort and imbalance during this time. In this section, we will explore herbs such as raspberry leaf, cramp bark, and ginger, which have been traditionally used to ease menstrual cramps, regulate cycles, and promote hormonal balance. We will also discuss the role of lifestyle factors such as diet, exercise, and stress management in supporting menstrual wellness and harmony.

Herbal Solutions for Pregnancy and Postpartum

Pregnancy and childbirth are profound experiences that require special care and support. In this section, we will explore herbs such as red raspberry leaf, nettle, and oatstraw, which have been traditionally used to nourish the body, support healthy fetal development, and prepare the uterus for labor. We will also discuss herbal remedies for common discomforts of pregnancy such as nausea, fatigue, and insomnia, as well as postpartum herbs for promoting recovery, lactation, and emotional well-being.

Balancing Hormones Throughout a Woman's Life

Hormonal balance is essential for women's health and vitality at every stage of life, from adolescence to menopause and beyond. In this section, we will explore herbs such as vitex, black cohosh, and dong quai, which have been traditionally used to support hormonal balance, ease symptoms of PMS and menopause, and promote overall well-being. We will also discuss the importance of addressing underlying imbalances and lifestyle factors in achieving hormonal harmony and optimal health.

As we explore these herbal remedies for women's health, let us remember the innate wisdom of the female body and the power of nature to nurture and support us throughout the various stages of life. By embracing the healing gifts of herbal medicine and honoring our bodies' natural rhythms and cycles, we can cultivate a deeper sense of vitality, balance, and empowerment as women.

Chapter 8: Herbal Remedies for Men's Health

Men's health encompasses a range of physical and emotional needs that are unique to their biology and life experiences. In this chapter, we will explore herbal remedies that support men's health and well-being, addressing concerns such as prostate health, vitality, and overall vitality.

Natural Support for Prostate Health

The prostate gland plays a crucial role in men's reproductive and urinary health, yet it is susceptible to enlargement and other conditions as men age. In this section, we will explore herbs such as saw palmetto, pygeum, and stinging nettle, which have been traditionally used to support prostate health, reduce inflammation, and alleviate symptoms of benign prostatic hyperplasia (BPH). We will also discuss lifestyle factors such as diet, exercise, and stress management that can contribute to prostate wellness and longevity.

Boosting Vitality and Stamina

Vitality and stamina are essential aspects of men's overall well-being, enabling them to thrive in their personal and professional lives. In this section, we will explore herbs such as ginseng, maca, and ashwagandha, which have adaptogenic properties that can enhance energy, endurance, and resilience to stress. We will also discuss the role of nutrition, exercise, and restorative practices such as meditation and deep breathing in promoting vitality and longevity.

Herbal Solutions for Men's Unique Health Needs

Men face a variety of health challenges throughout their lives, from cardiovascular disease and erectile dysfunction to mental health concerns such as depression and anxiety. In this section, we will explore herbs such as hawthorn, horny goat weed, and St. John's wort, which have been traditionally used to support heart health, sexual function, and emotional well-being in men. We will also discuss the importance of regular health screenings, preventive care, and open communication with healthcare providers in maintaining optimal health and wellness.

As we explore these herbal remedies for men's health, let us remember that true well-being encompasses not only physical health but also emotional, mental, and spiritual vitality. By embracing the healing gifts of herbal medicine and adopting holistic lifestyle practices, men can cultivate a deeper sense of vitality, resilience, and fulfillment in every aspect of their lives.

Chapter 9: Herbal Remedies for Children and Families

The health and well-being of children and families are paramount concerns for caregivers and parents. In this chapter, we will explore safe and effective herbal remedies that can support the health and vitality of

children and the whole family.

Safe and Gentle Herbs for Kids

Children have unique health

needs and sensitivities, making it

essential to choose herbs that are

safe and appropriate for their age

and development. In this section,

we will explore gentle herbs such as chamomile, lemon balm, and catnip, which are commonly used to soothe digestive discomfort, promote relaxation, and support restful sleep in children. We will also discuss practical considerations such as dosing, administration methods, and potential interactions with medications to ensure the safe use of herbal remedies for kids.

Natural Remedies for Childhood Ailments

From colds and coughs to earaches and teething pain, childhood ailments are common concerns for parents and caregivers. In this section, we will explore herbal remedies such as elderberry syrup, mullein garlic ear oil, and chamomile teething gel, which can help alleviate symptoms and support the body's natural healing processes. We will also discuss the importance of maintaining a healthy diet, promoting good hygiene practices, and fostering emotional resilience in children to prevent illness and promote overall well-being.

Integrating Herbal Medicine into Family Wellness

The health and wellness of a family extend beyond individual concerns to encompass the collective well-being of all its members. In this section, we will explore ways to integrate herbal medicine into the daily lives of families, from creating herbal first aid kits and home remedy cabinets to incorporating herbal teas, tinctures, and culinary herbs into meals and snacks. We will also discuss the importance of fostering a connection with nature, cultivating a supportive community, and modeling healthy lifestyle habits for children to promote holistic family wellness.

As we explore these herbal remedies for children and families, let us remember that nurturing health and well-being is a collaborative endeavor that requires love, patience, and compassion. By embracing the healing gifts of herbal medicine and fostering a culture of wellness within the family, caregivers and parents can empower their children to thrive and flourish in mind, body, and spirit.

Chapter 10: Cultivating Herbal Wisdom

Cultivating herbal wisdom is not just about acquiring knowledge; it's a journey of connection, stewardship, and empowerment. In this final chapter, we will explore practical ways to deepen your relationship with herbal medicine, from growing your own medicinal garden to advocating for herbal education in your community.

Growing Your Own Medicinal Garden

There is no greater joy for an herbalist than tending to a garden teeming with medicinal plants. In this section, we will explore the joys and challenges of growing your own medicinal garden, from selecting the right location and soil to choosing the best herbs for your climate and growing conditions. We will also discuss practical tips for planting, watering, harvesting, and preserving your herbs, as well as creative ways to incorporate them into your daily life for health and wellness.

Sustainable Practices in Herbalism

As stewards of the earth, it is our responsibility to harvest and utilize medicinal plants in a sustainable and ethical manner. In this section, we will explore sustainable practices in herbalism, from wildcrafting and cultivation to ethical sourcing and conservation. We will also discuss the importance of honoring indigenous knowledge, supporting small-scale herbal farmers, and advocating for policies that protect plant biodiversity and traditional healing practices.

Becoming an Herbal Advocate in Your Community

Herbal medicine has the power to transform lives and communities, but its potential can only be realized through education, advocacy, and collective action. In this section, we will explore ways to become an herbal advocate in your community, from sharing your knowledge and experiences with friends and family to volunteering with local herbal organizations and supporting herbal education initiatives. We will also discuss the importance of fostering partnerships with healthcare providers, policymakers, and other stakeholders to promote the integration of herbal medicine into mainstream healthcare systems.

As we conclude our journey through the world of herbal medicine, let us remember that herbal wisdom is not just a body of knowledge—it's a way of living in harmony with nature, embracing the healing gifts of the earth, and empowering ourselves to take charge of our health and well-being. By cultivating herbal wisdom in our own lives and sharing it with others, we can create a healthier, more vibrant world for generations to come.

Conclusion: Embracing the Herbal Lifestyle

As we come to the end of our exploration into the world of herbal medicine, we are reminded of the timeless wisdom encoded within the leaves, roots, and flowers of the natural world. Throughout this journey, we have delved into ancient traditions, rediscovered forgotten remedies, and empowered ourselves to embrace a more holistic approach to health and wellness.

Herbal medicine is not just about treating symptoms; it's about nurturing the body, mind, and spirit in harmony with the rhythms of nature. It's about recognizing the interconnectedness of all living beings and honoring the sacred bond between humanity and the plant kingdom.

As we reflect on the knowledge we have gained and the experiences we have shared, let us remember that true healing begins with a deep reverence for the earth and all its inhabitants.

By embracing the herbal lifestyle—cultivating medicinal gardens, practicing sustainable herbalism, and advocating for herbal education in our communities—we can create a world where health and vitality are accessible to all.

May we continue to walk this path of herbal wisdom with

humility, gratitude, and compassion, honoring the ancient traditions that have guided us and the future generations who will carry the torch of healing forward. And may we always remember that the greatest medicine of all is love—for ourselves, for each other, and for the magnificent world that sustains us.

As we bid farewell to this journey, let us carry the wisdom of the herbs in our hearts, allowing their gentle guidance to illuminate our path and inspire us to live each day with intention, vitality, and joy.

With blessings of health, happiness, and harmony,

Made in the USA
Coppell, TX
27 April 2024

31738894R20066